5-Minute
HAIRSTYLES

"To my children. May you always have the confidence to chase your dreams."

Published in 2016 by
HarperDesign
An Imprint of HarperCollinsPublishers
195 Broadway
New York, New York 10007
Tel: 212-207-7000
Fax: 855-746-6023
harperdesign@harpercollins.com
www.hc.com

Distributed throughout North America by
HarperCollins Publishers
195 Broadway
New York, New York 10007

ISBN 978-0-06-246684-6

Printed in China

Library of Congress Control Number to come.

First Printing, 2016

Publisher: Mark Searle
Editorial Director: Isheeta Mustafi
Commissioning Editor: Alison Morris
Editor: Angela Koo
Junior Editor: Abbie Sharman
Art Director: Michelle Rowlandson
Design concept: Michelle Rowlandson
Book layout: Agata Rybicka and Richard Peters
Cover design: Michelle Rowlandson
Photographer: Sara Bishop

Cover Credits:
Front (clockwise from top): Photographer Sara Bishop, stylist Jenny Strebe, model Angela Gutierrez; Getty Images; photographer Sara Bishop, stylist Jenny Strebe, model Alexia Poisot; photographer Sara Bishop, stylist Jenny Strebe, model Cheyenne Folkert.
Back (left to right): Photographer Sara Bishop, stylist Jenny Strebe, models Jacque Stuard, Jasmine Jacobson, Mallory Jarvis, Jasmine Jacobson.

5-Minute HAIRSTYLES

50 Super Quick 'Dos to Wear and Go

JENNY STREBE

HARPER DESIGN

An Imprint of HarperCollinsPublishers

CONTENTS

Double-plaited bun, pages 62-63

INTRODUCTION

Through the process of creating books and traveling to different salons for meet-and-greets, book signings, and classes, I have learned many valuable hair tricks. One of these tricks is the art of creating a great hairstyle in very little time. So, to share the benefits of my experience with you, I have interpreted my own hairstyles to come up with a collection of looks that can be created in under five minutes!

I created this book with a typical girl on the go in mind. Sometimes life gets crazy and you need a look that will fit your needs throughout the day. The one thing you want but just don't have is time. Well, that and a pair of comfortable heels! So whether you are heading to the beach with your girls, need a quick style for work, or are going out on a date, these hairstyles will get you out the door without an ounce of stress.

In the chapters that follow I have created tutorials that will teach you how to create the five-minute hairstyle of your choice in five easy steps. I've also included a few well-known favorites, to which I've added a touch of modern flair! But remember, what makes these looks so great is that there is plenty of room to add your own personal touch. Whether it's adjusting the style of braid you use, or adding a special accessory, you can make each of these styles your own—just focus on whatever looks good on you. So, follow the steps, get a feel for the possibilities, and then let your imagination run wild.

Happy styling!

Jenny Strebe

Double twists into simple plait,
pages 116-117

Ponytails

BRAIDED-HEADBAND PONY

Whether you're sporty, girly, or just need a little something extra to add to your everyday ponytail, the braided headband pony is a great quick fix! While ideal on mid-length to long hair, this look is doable on short hair with just a few more pins. You can also go from day to night by curling your ponytail and adding some shine spray. All you need is two hair elastics, a comb, and a bobby pin.

1. Separate a two- to three-inch-wide section of hair from behind one ear.

2. Divide this into three equal strands, then create a basic three-strand braid, taking the right strand over the middle, then taking the left strand over the new middle strand (originally the right strand), and so on.

3. Secure the end of the braid with an elastic. (You can also create fullness in your braid at this point by pulling on each section, as if you are fanning out a deck of cards.)

4. Bring the braid across the top of your head but do not pin it in place. Comb the rest of your hair back into a high ponytail.

5. Now hide the ends of the braid and the elastic by tucking them through the side of the ponytail. Pin this into place out of sight.

tip

If you are having trouble keeping the base of your braid nice and tight at the roots, then simply direct the sectioned-off hair upward and braid in that direction.

BOUFFANT PONY

This is a classic style with a modern twist. You can make this look as messy or as neat as you want, and in hardly any time at all. To make the ponytail more decorative, take a small one-inch section of hair from the ponytail and wrap it around the hair elastic. You can even braid the section before wrapping it if you want! The only tools you'll need are a duckbill clip, a comb, and a hair elastic.

1. Part out a triangular section of hair from above your brow arch and clip it away for later.

2. Now take horizontal sections of hair from behind this triangular section and aggressively tease each one until you reach where your head begins to curve down, a few inches above your nape.

3. Now drop all of the teased hair and lightly comb over the top of it to create a sleeker look on the surface.

4. Gather all of your hair (apart from the triangular section) to the back of your head and secure it with a hair elastic.

5. Finally, unclip the triangular section and swoop it over to the side as desired, tucking it behind your ear, and using a pin to secure it if necessary.

tip

When securing your ponytail with the elastic, be careful not to pull too tightly or you will lose volume in your bouffant.

FAKE LONG PONY

Fake the look of long and luscious locks easily with this five-minute hairstyle! You'll find that there are no limits to the occasions when you can wear this pony, and you can make it even more your own simply by adding accessories or curls. For this simpler version, you will need nothing more than a comb, some duckbill clips, and a couple of hair elastics to complete the look.

1. Take a horseshoe-shaped section from your low crown to the bottom of your ear on either side and tie or clip the top sections out of the way for now.

2. Now use a hair elastic to secure the lower section of hair into a low ponytail.

3. Next, release the top sections of hair and create a second ponytail a few inches above your first pony.

4. Lightly tease the base of both ponytails to create a fuller look.

5. To finish off, hold on to the base of the top ponytail and lightly pinch and pull the hair around your hairline to create a bit of extra fullness.

tip

This look works best on textured hair, since this will hide the bottom ponytail more effectively.

BRAID INTO PONY

This is a great style for those of you who have bangs and want to keep them out of your face. This look works for everyone, though—bangs or no bangs! It is quick to achieve with just a comb and a hair elastic, and it lasts all day long, making it perfect for yoga, or just for every day. You can also mix things up by trying a half-up half-down version (see the half-up rope-braid topknot on pages 64–65).

1. Divide your hair in half, separating the front from the back. Take a small section of hair from in front of one ear and divide this into three.

2. Start a "lace braid" with these sections (working the strands underhand rather than the usual overhand), feeding portions of hair into the strands on either side of the braid as you progress.

3. Continue your braid, working right to left until you reach your opposite ear. Then continue with a regular braid until you reach the ends.

4. Secure this with a hair elastic, then "pancake" your braid (pulling at sections of it) for fullness and texture.

5. Now pull all of your hair back into a high ponytail, incorporating the braid.

tip

For a fuller ponytail, start off by creating some waves or curls in your hair. You may also want to wrap a strand of hair around the elastic holding your pony (see right).

FULL FISHTAIL PONY

The full fishtail pony is a fun way to add volume and texture to your ponytail in just a few easy steps. The best thing about this hairstyle is that it looks great lived-in, so you don't have to worry about it getting a little messy throughout the day. Wear it from class to class, or at work all day. Grab two hair elastics, a comb, and texturizing spray and let's get started!

1. Create a high ponytail.

2. Divide this ponytail into two equal-sized sections. Now separate out a small strand of hair from the outside of the right section. This will pass up and over to become incorporated into the section of hair on the left. This action is then repeated on the left, with a small strand of hair taken from the far left, then passed up and over to join the right section. (See step 3 on page 36 for an additional view.)

3. Repeat until you reach your desired length of fishtail, then secure the end with an elastic.

4. Apply some texturizing spray, then pull at individual strands of the fishtail to create fullness.

5. For extra volume, grab the sides of the fishtail at the base of the ponytail and pull them outward simultaneously.

tip

If you want the style to have a high-ponytail effect, insert a few bobby pins into the base of the ponytail.

DOUBLE TOPSY TAIL PONY

This is a modest and graceful hairstyle. It is incredibly easy to dress up or down, enabling you to create styles for all occasions, from errands to parties, using just two hair elastics, a duckbill clip, and a comb! If you would like more of a challenge, braid the ends of the top topsy tail before pulling it through the bottom topsy tail for some subtle texture.

1. Divide your hair in half horizontally from ear to ear. Clip the top section out of the way for now.

2. Gather all the hair from the bottom section and, using a hair elastic, create a low ponytail at the nape of your neck.

3. Create a hole in the middle of the base of the ponytail, then pull your hair up, fold it back on itself, and thread it down through this hole. This creates your topsy tail.

4. Now release the top section and create a ponytail directly above the bottom ponytail. Then make a second topsy tail to sit above the previous one.

5. Finally, feed the hair from your top topsy tail down through the bottom topsy tail to complete the look.

tip

To create a fuller effect, lightly spritz each topsy tail with some texturizing spray and then gently pull the strands outward.

SLEEK WRAPPED PONY

The sleek wrapped pony is a classic wear-everywhere style, equally suited to dressed-up or casual looks. It is easiest to do on mid-length to long straight hair, but if your hair fits into a ponytail, then give it a try! A hair elastic, some serum, a bobby pin, and a comb are all you'll need. To make it fun and flirty, you can even braid the small section of hair first (as on page 24).

1. Part your hair neatly to the desired side.

2. Comb your hair and gather it tightly at the nape of your neck. Make sure there are no lumps or bumps, and use a bit of light serum to make sure you get rid of any flyaways.

   Hold the base of the ponytail firmly and secure it with a hair elastic. To keep your ponytail central you can try keeping your head parallel to the floor.

3. Now separate out a one-inch section of hair from the ponytail on the underside.

4. Wrap this small section neatly around the elastic. To secure it in place, loop the end of the sectioned-out hair around a bobby pin, and then push the pin under and into the base of the ponytail.

tip

If your hair is naturally curly, give it a sleeker look before you start. Towel-dry it, then blow-dry it straight down with a paddle brush.

BRAID-WRAPPED PONY

The braid-wrapped pony is a time-efficient style that's suitable for everyone. In just a few minutes you get a chic look with a flirty twist. This hairstyle can be worn casually or to a special event—it's completely adaptable. And the only items you'll need to achieve it are a comb, a hair elastic, and a few bobby pins.

1. Comb through all of your hair, making sure there are no knots in it. Pull all of your hair to the lower back of your head.

2. Secure your hair in place here with a hair elastic.

3. Separate out a one-inch section from the ponytail on its underside, then clip the remainder of the ponytail out of the way for now.

4. Now create a simple braid with this small section of hair, and secure it with a hair elastic.

5. Unclip the rest of the ponytail and then wrap the braid around the base of the hair elastic. Secure it in place using a bobby pin or two.

tip

If you have thin hair, pull and stretch out the sectioned-off braid before you wrap it around the elastic to create more fullness.

DOUBLE-PONY POUF

The double-pony pouf is a really quick and feminine hairstyle. It's perfect if you want to keep things simple. And, if you want to add a bit more texture and edge, you can always curl your hair prior to styling it. As with all of the styles in this book, the tools you'll need are minimal—a comb and a few hair elastics. That's it!

1. Separate out a small triangular section of hair from brow arch to brow arch, going back three or four inches from your hairline (depending on the density of your hair).

2. Create your first ponytail by securing this sectioned-out hair with an elastic.

3. While holding on to the base of the ponytail, pull the gathered strands forward to create your first pouf.

4. Now gather up the rest of your hair and create another ponytail, securing it with an elastic.

5. Hold on to the base of this second ponytail and pinch and pull the strands out as before to create volume and fullness with this second pouf.

tip

If your hair lacks volume and texture, you may find it helpful to tease both of your poufs prior to securing them with hair elastics.

TEXTURED PONY

This quick, cute hairstyle is great for everyday use, and you don't even need a comb—using your fingers to comb through your hair instead will help to create more natural texture. You can use your fingers to tease out your ponytail, too, if you want to create a little more volume and drama. Just grab a hair elastic and a curling iron and you'll be ready to start.

1. Start by adding some curls and texture to your hair by wrapping one- to two-inch sections of hair around your curling iron. Just a few strands here and there will be enough, although if you have time on your hands you can go as far as you like!

2. Next take small sections of hair and lightly tease them at the roots with your fingers.

3. Now gently comb your hair back with your fingers. It's very important not to brush out any texture or volume while you are doing this.

4. Create a high ponytail by gathering your hair toward the high-crown area, securing it with an elastic.

5. Finally, pinch and pull at your roots to create a bit more volume. Hold on to your ponytail while you do this so that you don't dislodge it.

tip

If you want to mix this style up in a hurry, try playing with different textures by adding more curls or adding a braid.

FAUXHAWK PONY

The fauxhawk pony offers you a great party style in a pinch. Created with a simple pulled-out Dutch braid feeding into a ponytail, this style will give you an edgy look in under five minutes! What's more, you can wear this look all night long without worrying about maintenance, since it still looks amazing when it's lived-in. All you need is a comb, a duckbill clip, and two hair elastics.

1. Separate out a triangular section of hair at your forehead. (Clip the rest of your hair out of the way, if it helps.)

2. Grab a one- to two-inch section at the top of the triangle and divide it in three for your braid.

3. Unlike the inverted look of a French braid, a Dutch braid sits above the hair—each side strand passes under the middle strand and then up (the reverse of the French over-and-down movement). Start braiding the triangular section, absorbing new strands of hair from either side, as for a French braid.

4. Continue with a regular braid for a few inches beyond the triangular section, secure it with an elastic, then stretch out your braid for the fauxhawk effect.

5. Gather everything up into a single ponytail.

tip

If you want to create an even larger fauxhawk effect, tease the hair in your triangular section prior to braiding it.

2

Braids

KNOTTED FRENCH BRAID

The knotted French braid is a beautiful style that works well with both classic and more edgy looks, and it is very easy to adapt for all sorts of events. If your hair is straight, you can leave it as it is, or you can add curls. If your hair is short, you can adapt the knotted French braid and make it a bun instead. Just grab a comb and a hair elastic, and let's get started.

1. Starting from your hairline above your forehead, separate out a section of hair (two or three inches) and then divide this section in two.

2. Cross one section over the other, then loop it under and through to create a knot. Pull both sides firmly to tighten the knot.

3. Now take two more sections from the hairline of your face and level with the top of your knot, and incorporate them into each of the strands emerging from the first knot. Now tie another knot.

4. Continue this process until you reach the nape of your neck, then tie knots with the remaining two strands to your desired length and secure the ends with an elastic.

5. Finish off by stretching and pulling the knots to create volume and texture.

tip

Silky hair can be prone to slipping out of the knots. Try adding texture before styling by applying mousse or sea-salt spray to damp hair and then blow-drying it.

SIDE FISHTAIL BUN

The side fishtail bun is a trendy spin on your everyday side bun. It's fun, flirty, and easier to do than you think. This hairstyle is perfect for second-day hair; texture is definitely your friend for this look! Wear it for a special occasion or out to lunch with friends. Before you begin, gather together a hair elastic, comb, bobby pins, and some hairspray.

1. Gather all your hair to the desired side, and create a ponytail by securing it with a hair elastic.

2. Divide your ponytail into two equal sections.

3. Take a small piece of hair from the far side of the right section of the ponytail and add it to the left section, then repeat with the other side. Continue crisscrossing in this way until you've created your fishtail, then secure the ends with an elastic.

4. Now wrap your fishtail braid around the hair elastic to create the bun and secure it in place with bobby pins.

5. To finish, gently pull at some small sections of hair (about a quarter of an inch) from the crown of your head, to give the style some softness.

tip

If your hair is fine, pulling and stretching the fishtail braid prior to creating your bun will give you a much fuller effect.

SIDE ROPE BRAID

If you've ever twirled or twisted your hair, then you know how to create a rope braid! It may look tricky, but it is actually one of the easiest styles in this book. It is a quick, elegant way to get that second-day hair out of your face, and requires nothing more than a comb and a hair elastic. If you don't want your rope braid to the side, then do it straight back or throw it up into a ponytail.

1. Start with "textured" hair (hair that hasn't been washed for a day or so is perfect!). Pull your hair over to the desired side.

2. Divide your hair into two equal sections. Take the section to the front and start twisting it clockwise (toward your face).

3. Now take that section up and over the back section. Your front section should now be at the back. Now twist the second section clockwise.

4. Pass this newly twisted section up over the other section, then continue this up-and-over process until you reach your desired length of braid. Secure it with an elastic.

5. To give your braid some extra volume and a lived-in look, lightly pinch and pull pieces out of both twisted portions.

tip

If your hair is extremely layered and prone to falling out of place, curl your hair first. Curls will blend in better with the rope braid.

TUXEDO BRAID

This is the perfect cherry-topper to a standard half-up half-down style. Taking the extra step is simple but looks like you've made a whole lot of effort, and who doesn't enjoy a hairstyle that looks harder than it is? Two hair elastics and a comb are all that you'll need, plus some texturizing spray if your hair is slippery. If you're a little more braid-savvy, you can try substituting a fishtail braid (see pages 18–19).

1. Separate out a large section of hair on top of your head using a horseshoe-shaped parting.

2. Divide this horseshoe section into three equal strands and use them to create a simple braid. Braid right down and secure the ends with an elastic.

3. Now "pancake" out the braid to make it fuller. Apply a texturizing spray if your hair is prone to slipping out of place.

4. Next, take a small strand of hair from in front of each ear but below the horseshoe section.

5. Take both of these sections and crisscross them over the braid. Then, holding the end of the braid up out of the way, connect the two sections with a hair elastic that will then be hidden underneath the hanging braid.

tip

If you want your hair to look fuller and longer, simply attach a few hair extensions for a more dramatic look.

STACKED SIDE BRAID

This quick tutorial offers a handy way to make your everyday side braid look a little bit more intricate. All you do is create two braids and then intertwine them with the help of a comb, a few hair elastics, and some bobby pins. This will result in a look that will take you effortlessly from poolside to happy hour out with your friends.

1. Divide your hair into two sections horizontally, with the bottom section denser than the top. Clip away the top section for later.

2. With the bottom section, create a standard braid on your desired side.

3. Secure the end of the braid with a hair elastic, then "pancake" the braid to create more volume and texture.

4. Now release the top section of hair and use it to create a tight braid right over the top of the lower braid. Secure the ends with another hair elastic.

5. Connect the top braid to the bottom braid by taking the end of the top braid and looping it through the bottom braid. Secure the two braids together with a bobby pin on the underside of the braids.

tip

If you fancy a looser, more feminine look, try leaving some strands of hair out of the braids and curling them.

TWIN-BRAID HALF-DOWN

This super-quick style is great for longer hair, and you'll need nothing more than a comb, a duckbill clip, and some hair elastics to complete it. The braids come together to create a classic and delicate look that you can switch up, depending on your mood. Wear this versatile look anywhere you want and embrace the compliments that will come your way!

1. Part your hair to the desired side. Take a triangular section of hair, two to three inches wide, from the right side of your head and create a braid. Once you are halfway down, clip the braid away for later, then repeat on the other side.

2. Take both braids to the back of your head and overdirect them toward your left side. Clip both braids together.

3. Now connect the braids by incorporating them both into a new braid. Secure the ends with a hair elastic.

4. Clip this first finished braid out of the way.

5. Now repeat steps 1 to 3, this time using sections taken from underneath the top braid and directed to the right instead of the left. Unclip the top section and place it over the bottom braid to finish.

tip

If you would like a longer braid, simply adding in some hair extensions before styling will give you an instant solution!

MILKMAID BRAID

This is the new messy bun—simple, stylish, and perfect for pool parties or hanging out with girlfriends. You can wear it effortlessly all day long, and the bonus is that it makes for great second-day hair once you take the braids out. It's best on long, unlayered hair, but if you have shorter hair, try a half-up half-down version. Grab a comb, two hair elastics, and some bobby pins and let's begin!

1. Divide your hair vertically into two equal sections.

2. Starting on the right side, create a simple braid, securing the end with a hair elastic, and then do the same on the left side of your head.

3. Take each braid and gently "pancake" each segment out. This will give your braids a fuller appearance.

4. Now take the right braid and drape it over the top of your head. Then do the same with the left braid.

5. Finally, use as many bobby pins as you need to secure both braids in place.

tip

To make this look a bit more formal, use a shine spray to get rid of any flyaways.

BOXER BRAIDS

Boxer braids are a great go-to look—they're perfect for keeping your hair out of your eyes at the gym, and then just as perfect for lunch with your girlfriends afterward. You can style this look on clean hair or second-day hair. Either way, this 'do is achieved in just a few minutes, and it will see you right through the day. Throw a comb and two hair elastics in your gym bag and you'll be set!

1. Divide your hair evenly in half down the center, then comb through it.

2. On the right side, separate out a triangular section at your hairline and divide it into three equal strands.

3. Begin your first braid by taking the right strand under and into the middle, then take the left strand under and into the middle. This reversal of the French-braid method will produce a Dutch braid, which sits out from the head. Incorporate hair into your sections on either side as you progress.

4. When you reach the nape of your neck, continue with a regular Dutch braid until you reach the ends, then secure them with an elastic.

5. Repeat for the left-hand braid.

tip

If your hair is prone to flyaways then dampen it prior to starting. This will also help to create tighter braids.

DUTCH SIDE BRAID

As mentioned earlier, Dutch braids are similar to French braids in terms of technique, but with the Dutch braid sitting above the hair, it is a lot easier to make the style your own. You can also add volume by pulling on the strands, or add texture by teasing your roots before braiding. This style is ideal for long and medium-thick hair. Have a hair elastic and a comb on hand before starting!

1. Part your hair to the desired side. Take a section from the top and then divide it into three strands.

2. Start your braid by taking the right strand under and into the middle, then taking your left section under and into the middle.

3. Now begin feeding small sections of hair into the braid. Incorporate a one-inch section into the left strand and bring it under and into the middle. Then do the same with the right strand, and so on.

4. When all your hair has been incorporated, continue braiding to the end of your hair, and tie it with an elastic.

5. "Pancake" the individual strands to create a fuller-looking braid.

tip

If your hair is fine and you want a fatter braid, try blow-drying your hair with a texturizing or sea-salt spray prior to braiding.

LOW ROPE BRAID

Why not try giving your everyday braid a twist with this quick alternative? You can wear this versatile hairdo anywhere—to work or to the beach—and it has the bonus of highlighting any contrasting tones in your hair. The best part? Keep it clean or a little messy—either looks great! You'll need nothing more than a comb and two hair elastics to create it.

1. Comb your hair to your low nape and secure it in place with a hair elastic.

2. Now divide the hair of the ponytail into two equal strands.

3. Begin by twisting the right strand in a clockwise direction a few times.

4. Now take the twisted right strand up and over the left so that the left strand is now on the right. Repeat the previous step, this time twisting the new right strand clockwise and taking it up and over the other strand. When twisting your two sections together you should be working in a counterclockwise direction.

5. Repeat this process until you've reached your desired length, then secure the ends of the braid with a hair elastic.

tip

You can easily make this look your own by changing the location of the rope braid, or by adding more texture.

MERMAID-STYLE DOUBLE BRAID

This hairstyle is great for those of you with long, thick hair. It's a beautiful look for a date or just hanging out with friends. And best of all, it looks a whole lot harder than it is! As with all of the styles in this book, all you require are everyday tools—a duckbill clip, a couple of hair elastics, bobby pins, and a comb. You can also mix up the two different braids to better fit your personal style.

1. Divide your hair in half horizontally; the top section should be a little smaller than the bottom. Clip the top section out of the way for now.

2. Create a simple three-strand braid with the bottom section and secure it with an elastic.

3. Now release the top section and use it to create a fishtail braid (see page 18). Secure it with another elastic.

4. Next, flip the top braid up out of the way, and "pancake" the bottom braid by stretching the sections out aggressively. This will create extra volume.

5. To finish, tuck the end of the fishtail into the lower braid. To prevent the top braid from slipping out, lift both braids and secure the end of the fishtail from behind by weaving a bobby pin through from the back.

tip

If your hair is silky and prone to slipping out of braids, simply apply a texturizing spray or a dry shampoo before starting.

3

Buns

FAUX-FRINGE TOPKNOT

If you don't have bangs and you're unsure about whether to get them, the faux-fringe topknot will give you the perfect trial run. This hairstyle will have you out the door in less than five minutes, with a whole new do—and all the benefits of bangs without the commitment! All you'll need is a comb and some hair elastics, although you can make this fun and flirty by adding a jeweled headband.

1. Start by gathering your hair into a high ponytail. Secure it with a hair elastic.

2. Now create the basis for your faux fringe by folding the ponytail over so that its ends are pointing down toward your face.

3. Secure the loop formed in the ponytail in the previous step by attaching another hair elastic at the base of the fold.

4. Now gently spread the looped hair out evenly, which should result in a fuller, more fanned-out bun.

5. Finally, comb the hair that was left out of the loop forward to create your faux fringe.

tip

If your hair is really straight after creating the faux fringe, try using a flat iron to create a more natural bend.

TWIST-AND-TUCK BUN

This flirty summer look comes together in no time at all. We've used a floral headband, but you can easily dress this look down with a simpler design. Just make sure your band extends all the way round your head. (This one has ties at the back.) For an even more effortless look, leave some strands hanging loose and curl them. Best of all? A headband and some pins are all you'll need!

1. Pick out your favorite headband and secure it on your head. Make sure the headband is on top of your hair, not underneath it.

2. Now take two small strands (two to three inches) from just above each ear and twist them away from your face.

3. Begin to tuck the ends into your headband. The closer you tuck them into the band, the tighter the finished bun will be.

4. Continue taking small sections and tucking them into your headband. Pull on the sections if you want to make the tucks look a bit fuller.

5. When all your hair has been incorporated, secure the twists with a few bobby pins. If you have more layers, you may need a few extra bobby pins!

tip

Make sure to pick out a headband that fits you well. This will make it easier for the headband to hold the hair securely in place.

DOUBLE-BRAIDED BUN

The double-braided bun is a sexy and bold hairstyle. Ideal for long hair, this showstopping style only takes a few minutes to create. To make it even more edgy, tease the roots of your hair for added volume. Leave some strands of hair down for a more casual vibe, or curl the loose strands for a special occasion. You will need four hair elastics, a few bobby pins, and some hairspray.

1. Divide your hair in half horizontally, from ear to ear.

2. Comb the bottom section of hair into a low ponytail. A few inches above the bottom ponytail, comb the second section into a mid-ponytail.

3. Create a simple three-strand braid with the bottom ponytail and secure the ends with an elastic. Do the same with the top ponytail.

4. Now "pancake" each braid to create a disheveled, more textured look.

5. To finish, wrap the top braid around the elastic at the base of the braid. Pin it in place with bobby pins. Repeat this process for the bottom braid, then give everything a light mist of hairspray.

tip

To create a lighter feel, massage around the hairline with the palms of your hands after you have created your bun. This will give your hair a softer, more uneven texture.

HALF-UP ROPE-BRAID TOPKNOT

This topknot is perfect for those of you who struggle with keeping long hair out of your face. It is a great twist on the typical topknot, achieved with very little extra effort! The best thing about this look is that you can vary the braids to suit your mood and personal style. And all you'll need are minimal tools—two hair elastics, a duckbill clip, a few bobby pins, and a comb.

1. Separate your hair horizontally from ear to ear. Clip the lower section out of the way for now.

2. Comb the top section of hair toward the high-crown area and secure it in place with a hair elastic.

3. Divide this ponytail into two equal sections. Create a twist by following steps 3 and 4 on page 52, and secure the twist with an elastic when you've reached your desired length.

4. Holding on to the end of your rope braid, pinch and pull at random sections of it, tugging them in the direction of the base of the ponytail, to create a thicker appearance.

5. Now release your lower section of hair, then take your thickened rope braid, wrap it around the hair elastic, and secure it with bobby pins.

tip

Depending on how thick your hair is, you can include more or less hair in your ponytail to create a fatter or smaller topknot.

BRAIDED BUN

You can never go wrong with this effortless, classic style. Wear it to mask your second-day hair, or create a clean and formal look after a fresh wash. Either way, these five steps will have your hair looking amazing in no time! Make sure you have a comb, a couple of hair elastics, and a bunch of bobby pins on hand before you start.

1. Comb through your hair thoroughly and then gather it all at the nape of your neck to create a low ponytail.

2. Secure the pony with a hair elastic, making sure the rest of your hair remains smooth.

3. Divide the ponytail into three equal sections and create a simple three-strand braid, securing it at the end with another elastic.

4. Now "pancake" the braid a bit to create more fullness.

5. Finish by wrapping the braid around the base of the ponytail to create your braided bun. Pin it in place in a circular pattern using as many bobby pins as you need to hold it securely.

tip

If you're creating this look for a special occasion, try curling your hair before styling to give it a bit of extra interest and flair.

BOUFFANT INTO BACK BUN

This is another classic look that can be achieved in mere minutes and will keep your hair up and out of your face all day! Teasing your roots a little and then adding a few twists results in a demure style that is perfect for work or a stylish brunch. As always, tools are very simple—you will just need a comb, duckbill clips, and a few bobby pins.

1. Start by separating out a large section of hair on top of your head, from the forehead back to your high crown.

2. Keep the lower section out of the way for now with a clip or two. Meanwhile, working on your upper section, take one-inch portions and begin aggressively teasing the roots. Continue teasing until you've achieved your desired volume.

3. Now brush this whole section of hair out with your fingers while also pulling the hair back and forming a twist. Bobby pin it in place.

4. Release the lower section of hair, twist it from the roots to the ends, then create a low bun. Secure this with pins.

5. To add a bit more fullness, hold on to your bun and lightly pull on the bouffant.

tip

Teasing can make your hair prone to flyaways, so use a shine spray if this is a problem for your hair.

TWISTED TOPKNOT

Stay cute and flirty all day long with the twisted topknot! Whether you are having a lazy day or are a girl on the go, this is the perfect way to get your hair out of your face with minimal effort. If you want to make this look more fun, try it half-up half-down, and then curl the hair that hangs free for a more formal look. A hair elastic, a few bobby pins, and a comb are all you'll need on hand.

1. Comb your hair back tightly and up into your high-crown area.

2. Secure your hair into a high ponytail using a hair elastic.

3. Now pull this ponytail directly up and, holding it taut, twist it from the roots to the ends.

4. Give your twist some extra bulk and texture by grabbing bits of hair from the twist and pulling them down toward the base of the ponytail.

5. Finish off the look by creating a bun. Take the twisted ponytail and wrap it around the hair elastic, and then secure it in place with a handful of bobby pins.

tip

If your hair lacks texture, "grit" it up by using a texturizing spray first. This will give your bun a more consistent and longer-lasting fullness.

FORMAL TOP BUN

Once you've mastered this classic, you'll have a go-to look for dates, weddings, and everything in between! As glamorous as it looks, it can be created with just a few simple moves. Creating the curls may take a while to begin with, but you will soon be whipping them up in no time. You will need a comb, curling iron, some hair elastics, bobby pins, and hairspray.

1. Gather your hair up into a high-crown ponytail and secure it with a hair elastic.

2. Take a portion of hair from the ponytail and curl it from the roots to the ends, leaving it on the curling iron for a few seconds. If you have plenty of time and want a more intricate look, select a one- to two-inch section. Grab a larger section if you only have five minutes.

3. Carefully release the curl from the curling iron, maintaining its curl, and pin it in place. Curls should be arranged to form a bun.

4. Continue this technique, pinning curled sections around your elastic until all your hair has been curled. (Or save time if you like by opting to leave some strands hanging loose outside the bun.)

5. Make sure everything is held firmly with pins, then spray the bun with hairspray to finish.

tip

This is a great style whether you have bangs or not! If you do, you can either pin them back, or curl them and leave them down.

TRIPLE MESSY BUN

The triple messy bun will give you a super-cool twist on your day-to-day messy bun. This casual look is done in minutes but it can be worn all day long—it's meant to be messy, so there is no need to worry about trying to keep it perfectly in place throughout the day. As usual, simple tools are all you'll need: hair elastics, bobby pins, and a comb.

1. Take a small horseshoe-shaped section from the top of your head, with the parting reaching back to the crown area. Create a ponytail by securing the hair with a hair elastic.

2. Clip away your first ponytail for now, then take a horizontal section of hair from ear to ear to create a second ponytail. The third ponytail can then be created with the hair remaining below this.

3. Now take the first ponytail and tightly twist it from the base to the ends. Create a topknot bun by wrapping the twist around the base of the elastic.

4. Bobby pin the first bun in place, then create topknots in the same way with the remaining two ponytails.

5. For the final touch, pinch and pull each bun out gently to create a messier, fuller look.

tip

If you have straight hair that lacks fullness and texture, just add some curls before starting.

KNOTTED BACK BUN

The knotted back bun is a
trendy new way to make a
bun. It's fun, flirty, and
totally different. Wear this
to a concert or just out and
about—like so many styles
in this book, it's a look that
is totally versatile. And, of
course, it can be created in
no time at all. Grab a couple
of hair elastics, a comb, and
a few bobby pins and give it
a go!

1. Gather your hair at the back
   of your head and create a
   ponytail. Secure it firmly with
   a hair elastic.

2. Comb out the ponytail and
   then divide the hair into two
   equal sections.

3. Now take these two sections of
   hair and tie them into a knot.

4. Continue tying the two
   sections of hair into knots
   until you reach the ends,
   then secure the knotted braid
   you've created with an elastic.

5. Finally, wrap the knotted braid
   around the base of the ponytail
   to create a bun, and use bobby
   pins to hold it firmly in place.

tip

If you fancy more of an effortless,
bohemian style, take the knotted
braid and gently rub it between the
palms of your hands before you
create the bun.

LOW SNAKE-COIL BUN

This chic style looks good on everyone and yet it requires hardly any effort at all. In fact, lots of women coil their hair up into a snake-coil bun without even realizing that's what they're doing! The only items you'll need are a few hair elastics, a comb, some bobby pins, and some hairspray, but do feel free to spice this look up with some hair accessories if the mood calls for it.

1. Comb your hair back evenly to the nape of your neck.

2. Secure this low ponytail with a hair elastic.

3. Now twist the ponytail from the base to the tip as tightly as possible in order to create your snake coil.

4. Let the twist naturally coil around your hair elastic to create a bun and then use bobby pins to hold it in place. Use three to four bobby pins distributed evenly around the bun for maximum support.

5. Finish off by applying a bit of hairspray and then very gently comb through to get rid of any flyaways and create a sleeker look at your roots.

tip

If your hair is naturally curly or wavy, you can get a sleeker finish by round-brushing or flat-ironing your hair before you begin.

LOW BUN WITH BRAIDED HEADBAND

The low bun with braided headband is a boho-chic way to deal with that second-day hair, and one that, with practice, only takes a few minutes. Wear it casually or for a formal event—everyone will love how it looks, and you'll love how little time it takes to create! Simply grab a few hair elastics, a comb, and a handful of bobby pins and you'll be ready to begin.

1. Grab a two- to three-inch section of hair from behind one ear.

2. Now use this section to create a simple braid and secure the end with a hair elastic. Repeat steps 1 and 2 on the other side of your head.

3. Gather the rest of your hair to the nape of your neck and use a hair elastic to form a ponytail.

4. Twist the ponytail you have just created to form a bun, and then secure it firmly in place using a few bobby pins.

5. The last step is to bring the right and left braids over your head to create the braided headband. Tuck the ends of each braid into your hair to conceal them, and pin them in place.

tip

Get creative with your braids! See if you can find ways of making this style your own by mixing it up a bit and using different types of braid.

BRAID-WRAPPED TOPKNOT

The braid-wrapped topknot is a real classic. Not only is this style simple to create, it is also easy to morph from casual to special occasion, which is what makes it such a lasting favorite. This quick and efficient 'do can be rocked from the beach to the dance floor in just a few quick moves! Grab a comb, two hair elastics, a duckbill clip, and a few bobby pins, and let's get started.

1. Gather all of your hair into the high-crown area and secure it in place with a hair elastic.

2. Depending on how thick your hair is, take a one to two-inch section of hair from the ponytail you've just created and clip it out of the way for now.

   Twist the rest of the ponytail from roots to ends and wrap it around the hair elastic to create a topknot (see pages 78-79).

3. Secure the topknot in place with bobby pins.

4. Now take the sectioned-off hair and create a simple three-strand braid, securing the end with a hair elastic. Wrap the braid around the base of your topknot and secure it further with some more bobby pins.

tip

If you don't have hair long enough to wrap around your topknot, use a hair extension and braid it to create the braid instead.

4

Party Updos

ROPE-BRAID UPDO

The rope-braid updo is a wonderful style to master—with the help of just a comb, some clips, hair elastics, and bobby pins, a few simple twists will set you up for an amazing night out in just minutes! You can also downplay this look and create a more bohemian effect by pulling out the twists in the rope braid, or by leaving some strands out of the braid altogether.

1. Section out some hair at the back of your head from the crown to mid-ear, then clip the top sections out of the way.

2. Create a low ponytail, then begin your rope braid. Divide the pony into two equal sections. Twist the right section clockwise, then bring it up and over the left section (see page 52). Repeat this process until you have your desired length of braid.

3. Now wrap your rope braid around the elastic to create a bun and secure it with pins.

4. Release the clip on one side of your head and divide this section in half to create another rope braid. Secure it with an elastic, then repeat on the other side.

5. Drape one side braid over and around your bun and pin it in place, then do the same with the other side braid.

tip

When braiding the sides, twist them away from your face and then intertwine the sections in the opposite direction to the one that you twisted them in.

TOPSY TAIL TUCK ROLL

The topsy tail tuck roll is an elegant, discreet hairstyle that flatters everyone. Wear it to a party or on a date—either way, you are bound to attract attention! This style works best on mid-length, medium to thick hair, but it suits all ages, and you can add some glamour simply by using sparkly hair accessories. You will need some hairspray, a comb, a hair elastic, and bobby pins to create this.

1. Begin by pulling your hair back into a low ponytail and securing it with an elastic.

2. Separate the hair at the base of the ponytail, just above your hair elastic, to create a small hole. Lift the ponytail up and pass it through this hole, pulling it through completely. This action will cause the sides of your hair to roll inward, creating a topsy tail effect.

3. Now prepare a roll by wrapping the pony around the index and middle fingers of one hand until you have a shape you are happy with.

4. Hold the roll firmly in place with one hand while you use your free hand to secure it with plenty of pins.

5. Finish by combing down any flyaways and using hairspray to keep everything in place.

tip

If you have naturally straight hair, curl it prior to starting to help limit any flyaways.

TWIST-AND-TEASE LOW UPDO

The twist-and-tease low updo is the perfect look for a date—it takes under five minutes to do and can easily be dressed up or down by changing out hair accessories. For example, try rocking this look during the day by going for a boho effect with some fake flowers or a floral headband. Otherwise, the basics you'll need are a comb, duckbill clips, some bobby pins, and a hair elastic.

1. Begin by taking a section of hair running from your crown to mid-ear. Clip the upper sections to either side, out of the way for now.

2. Now create a low ponytail by gathering the hair at the nape of your neck and securing it with a hair elastic.

3. Next, create your twist-and-tease effect by aggressively twisting your ponytail from the base through to the ends.

4. Wrap this twisted hair around the base of the hair elastic to create a bun, and secure it in place with some bobby pins.

5. Now release your side sections from their clips. Twist both of these sections using the same technique as before, and then drape the pieces over the bun. Pin them in place.

tip

If your hair is very thick, feel free to section out smaller pieces for your twists.

PULLED-OUT BRAIDED UPDO

The sophistication and detail of this look make it striking enough to wear to an important event, and you'll be amazed when you discover just how easy it is to create. You can also give it a more edgy look by teasing your hair prior to styling, and by pulling hair out of the braid more vigorously. Make sure you have a comb, a few bobby pins, and a hair elastic on hand before you start.

1. Working from the temples back to the crown of the head, take a horseshoe-shaped section of hair.

2. Divide this into three equal strands. Start creating a Dutch braid by taking the right strand under and into the middle, then take the left strand under and into the middle.

3. Now incorporate a one-inch section of hair into the right strand before bringing it under and into the middle. Repeat on the left side. Continue in this way until all your hair is incorporated, then continue the braid to the ends. Secure it with an elastic.

4. Stretch out the braid vigorously to create volume and texture.

5. Finish by creating your bun. Flip the braid under and then pin it in place, arranging it in a rounded shape.

tip

If you decide to create a looser braid by pulling the strands out farther, make sure you anchor the bun well with bobby pins for longer-lasting fullness.

LOW FLOWER UPDO

If you know how to create a simple three-strand braid then you will be able to create the low flower updo. This is yet another hairstyle that looks more complicated than it is—and who doesn't love that? If your hair is dirty and you're in a pinch, do this look to the side and then throw on a hat or a headband. Grab a comb, a hair elastic, and some bobby pins and let's work through the steps!

1. Begin by combing your hair toward the back of your head and secure it with a hair elastic.

2. Now divide the ponytail you've just created into three strands to create a simple braid.

3. When you reach the end of the braid, secure it with an elastic. Then, while holding on to the braid from one side, pull and stretch out the opposing side to create volume. Do this down the length of the braid.

4. Take the side of the braid that hasn't been stretched out and wrap it tightly around the base of your pony. The stretched-out half of the braid should be sitting around the outside of the bun, creating your "flower."

5. Secure your braid in place using bobby pins, maintaining a circular shape all the way around for the most realistic flower effect.

tip

If there are any straight ends of hair left out of the elastic once you've created your bun, try curling them so that they bend naturally around the flower.

STACKED-TWISTS UPDO

If you're heading out and you're facing a time crunch, then look no further than the stacked-twists updo! Make this look formal or casual by starting out with either clean or textured hair. This look involves nothing more than a few easy twists, and you can really make it your own by embellishing it with accessories. Otherwise all you need is a comb and a few bobby pins.

1. Part your hair on the desired side, then separate a horizontal section on one side (one to two inches), working back from your hairline.

2. Twist this section of hair away from your face while directing it behind and toward the other side of your head.

3. Pin the twist in place.

4. Now take an equal-sized section from the other side of your head and repeat steps 2 and 3. Continue working your horizontal sections from right to left in the same way. Keep going until you have incorporated all the hair on both sides and have just a few strands remaining at the nape of your neck.

5. Take the very ends of the leftover strands, twist them, and then pin them into the rest of the updo.

tip

This look is easily transformed into a half-up half-down style. Once you have your desired number of twists, simply leave the remaining hair down. The result will be something like step 4.

SIDE-KNOT UPDO

Heading out with just five minutes to spare? Not a problem—needing just a comb, a hair elastic, and a few bobby pins, the side-knot updo gives you a quick and handy way to switch up a traditional side braid. The knotted effect adds an interesting texture for no extra effort. If you want a more formal look, simply curl your hair, do the knot to the back, and spritz on some shine spray.

1. Comb your hair to the desired side and then divide it into two equal sections.

2. Cross one section over the other, then pull it under and through the gap between them to create a simple knot.

3. Continue with this knotting technique until you've reached your desired length. When you're finished, secure the end of the braid with a hair elastic.

4. Now take the end of your knotted braid. Loop it around and then tuck it neatly inside the initial division of hair you made in step 1.

5. Finish by pinning the loop securely in place.

tip

If you want more volume in your updo, tease the roots of your hair prior to starting.

5

Down Styles

HALF-DOWN TWISTED TOPSY TAIL

The half-down twisted topsy tail is a quick style for a chic girl on the go. Wear the version shown here for errands, or curl it before heading out on that hot date—either way, this style will leave you looking and feeling great! You can even braid the topsy tail if you want to take things a step further. Best of all, a comb and a hair elastic are all you'll need to achieve this look.

1. Start by dividing your hair in half horizontally, parting it from ear to ear.

2. Now comb the top section into a ponytail and secure it with a hair elastic.

3. Divide this hair evenly in half at the base of the ponytail.

4. Take the ponytail and bring it up and down through the center of the halved hair at the base. Pull the ponytail down and all the way through.

5. Finally, to exaggerate the twist and create a fuller look, carefully pull out small sections of the topsy tail.

tip

If your hair is extremely fine and you want to rock this 'do, lightly curl your hair prior to styling. This will help add volume.

CURLY FRONT TWIST

This is a fun and fresh alternative to a French braid. Using a similar technique, you add strands of hair into your twist. However, using only two strands of hair instead of three makes it a much easier choice if you are unsure of how to braid, or only have limited time! You'll need a comb, some hair elastics, a couple of bobby pins, a duckbill clip, and a curling iron.

1. Part your hair to the desired side. Grab a small section at the front (two to three inches) and create your first twist.

2. Take another small section of hair directly under the first one and incorporate it into the first twist. Twist it a couple of times. This will give the twist a better ridge at the hairline.

3. Continue incorporating new sections of hair into the twist until you reach your ear, then continue twisting the hair through to the ends. Clip this against your head for now.

4. Take a small section of hair from above where you would like to pin your twist and clip it out of the way. Pin the twist in place, then release the hair on top to conceal the pin.

5. Finish by using your curling iron to add a quick curl or two if you want extra volume.

tip

If you have layers in your hair, or a lot of flyaways, try using a little pomade to keep the twist looking neat and fresh.

POMPADOUR

Although you will learn how to complete this 'do in hardly any time at all, the pompadour is one of the most diverse looks around. Wear it out on a date or with your best girls—with a little hair product and some back-combing, you'll be ready to rock your evening! Gather together a comb, a few duckbill clips, some hairspray, and a hair elastic, and let's work through the process step by step.

1. Begin by separating out a triangular section of hair at the top of your head and clip it out of the way for now.

2. Take a section from just above your right ear and do the same on your left side, gather these sections into the low-crown area and create a ponytail by securing them both together with an elastic. Be sure to keep the sides smooth and tight.

3. Release the top triangular section and use your comb to tease your hair at the roots until you have created your desired volume.

4. Now lightly comb over the top of your hair to cover up the teasing.

5. Finally, add some hairspray and comb through the sides to create a sleeker look.

tip

If your hair is thick and heavy, use a few bobby pins to help maintain the volume.

BOUFFANT WITH BRAIDED HEADBAND

While there are many hairstyles that should remain in the 1970s, this inspired look is not one of them. The braids add a flirty modern twist, and the volume at the crown of your head can be as dramatic or as restrained as you like. You also have the option of curling your hair or leaving it straight. All you need is a duckbill clip, two hair elastics, some bobby pins, and a comb.

1. Take a two-inch section from directly behind one ear and clip the rest of your hair out of the way for now.

2. Create a simple braid with the small section, then secure it with an elastic. If you want to keep the braid lying flat against the head, overdirecting it upward while you work will help. Create a matching braid on the other side.

3. Take a vertical section of hair, a couple of inches from your hairline, and tease aggressively at the roots.

4. Continue back-combing vertical sections of hair in this way until you've achieved the desired volume.

5. Now drape each braid across your head, about an inch from your hairline, and secure them behind the ears with pins.

tip

If your hair is resistant to back-combing, create a better hold by adding some dry shampoo to the roots before you begin.

TEASE AND TIE

As long as you have hair long enough to tie into a knot, then you can accomplish this awesome look! This is one of the easiest styles you can choose, and it's perfect for when you fancy an unfussy, casual look. You simply tease your hair at the roots with a comb, add a bit of hairspray or texturizing spray, then tie two strands of hair together behind your head.

1. Working from the high crown to the low crown, take small sections of hair and tease the roots of each one in turn.

2. When the teasing is complete, lightly comb over the top of it to create a clean-textured layer of hair on the surface.

3. Now grab a one- to two-inch section from above your ear on both sides of your head.

4. Bring these two sections of hair to the back of your head, and tie them together in the low-nape area. Tie a second knot underneath the first knot.

5. To give a little bit of extra security, attach a hair elastic underneath both knots to hold them in place.

tip

If you have silky hair, add a pomade to the side sections prior to tying. This will help the style last all day!

SIDESWEPT PINBACK

The sideswept pinback is a great style on everyone and on all hair lengths, and with only a few simple steps, you'll be on your way out the door in less than five minutes. Like many of the other styles in this book, this is an incredibly versatile look, too—keep it casual for work, or glamorous for a night out! All you need to have on hand is a comb, a curling iron, a hair clip, and a bobby pin or two.

1. Prep your hair before styling by working through any tangles you may have and adding a light curl with your curling iron. You don't need to spend much time on this—just a few strands is fine.

2. Part your hair to the desired side, working from your hairline down to the nape of your neck.

3. Clip the larger section out of the way for now.

4. Take the smaller section of hair and twist it toward the far side of your neck. Secure this hair in place using a bobby pin.

5. Now release the clipped-away section of hair. Re-curl any strands that may have loosened too much in the meantime, and then finish off the whole look with hairspray.

tip

You can change this whole look just by the way you prep your hair prior to styling. For a casual look, go with straight hair, or add glamour with tight curls.

TWIST AND PUSH-UP STYLE

Not only can this classic hairstyle be created in minutes, it can also be worn anywhere and everywhere. You can tease your roots and curl your hair before you begin styling for a more formal look, or you can begin with natural hair if you want to keep it looking modest and minimal for everyday wear. You will need just a comb and a few bobby pins to hold everything in place.

1. Part your hair if desired and then divide your hair in half horizontally, from ear to ear.

2. Pull your hair back toward the low-crown area, then begin rotating the hair with your hand, creating a slight French twist.

3. Now push the twisted hair upward so that you create more volume in the crown.

4. Secure the twist in place with a few bobby pins. On the right side of the twist, grab the hair with the lip of a pin, then rotate and push the pin into the twist, directing it upward.

5. Add just a bit more volume and texture to finish off by gently holding on to the base of your twist while you pull carefully at the hair around the top of your head.

tip

If you have thin hair, or you just don't want to back-comb, try blow-drying with a volumizing mousse before starting.

DOUBLE TWISTS INTO SIMPLE BRAID

This five-minute style is great for summer, and you can make it as simple or as complicated as you want. For instance, instead of twisting your hair, you could simply braid it. This hairstyle is ideal for those of you with minimal layering in your hair, but if you do have a lot of layers, simply curl before starting. You'll need a hair elastic, a duckbill clip, and a comb on hand before you begin.

1. On each side of your head, separate out a large triangular section (around two or three inches wide).

2. Twist the hair in each triangular section away from your face and down at an angle, toward the lower back of your head.

3. Connect both twists at the back and clip them together for later. Now divide all of your hair into three equal sections. Keeping the twists clipped together, create a three-strand braid, incorporating the hair emerging from the twists.

4. Braid your hair until you reach the ends, then secure them with a hair elastic.

5. Finish off by removing the clip from the twists, then "pancake" the braid to create more fullness.

tip

For a more textured and bohemian look, create this style on naturally curly or previously curled hair.

6

Resources

TOOLS

Blow-dryer
A styling tool that, in addition to drying hair, is great for adding volume or for smoothing and straightening out hair.

Bobby pins
These are used to hold sections of hair in place. (For larger sections of hair, such as buns, you can also use longer hair pins, rather than bobby pins.)

Curling iron
A styling tool that uses heat to create a consistent curl on a portion of hair.

Dry shampoo
A hairstyling product that helps give greasy or second-day hair a freshly washed look. It is also a good product for adding texture to hair before styling.

Duckbill clip
This is a large hair clip used to hold sections of hair out of the way while you work on another section.

Flat iron
A styling tool that uses heat between two metal plates in order to take hair from curly to straight.

Hair elastic
A rubber band that gathers and secures hair in the form of a ponytail. It is also used to secure the ends of the hair—for example, with braids.

Hair extension
Synthetic or real human hair woven together on a hair weft that you can attach to your own natural hair to add length or volume. There are several different types of extensions for temporary use that can be attached using glue or tape, protein bonded, or clipped in.

Paddle brush
A flat brush that can be used to detangle, straighten, and flatten hair. It can also be used to tame flyaways.

Pomade
A water-based substance that is used to style hair and set styles. It does not dry out the hair and leaves it looking shiny and slick.

Serum
A thicker shine product that helps with flyaways.

Shine spray
A product that adds shine to frizzy hair.

Texturizing spray
A product that adds texture to the hair.

Volumizing mousse
Also referred to as styling foam, this product is used to give the hair more volume and shine. It is often used while blow-drying the hair.

Low bun with braided headband variation, pages 80-81

GLOSSARY

Back-combing
A technique that uses a comb to reverse-brush the hair (in the direction of the roots) in order to create long-lasting volume. (Also known as "teasing.")

Braid
Also referred to as a plait, a technique that involves weaving sections of hair into each other. There are several ways you can braid your hair, including three-strand braids, French braids, and fishtail braids.

Crown
The upper back portion of your head.

Dutch braid
A three-strand technique that crosses sections under one another, while also drawing hair in from either side of the braid in turn. Similar to a French braid, but in this case the resulting braid sits on top of the hair.

Fishtail braid
A two-strand technique that crisscrosses small strands of hair alternately, overlapping two larger sections, to create a thick braid with a densely woven appearance.

French braid
A three-strand technique that crosses sections of hair over one another, while also incorporating hair from either side of the braid. Unlike the Dutch braid, the French braid has an inverted appearance, due to the over-and-under movement of the strands.

High crown
The highest point of the crown on the back of the head.

Hairline
The hair that grows along the perimeter of your head, including around your face and along your neckline.

Hair section
A section of hair that is clipped back while you work on other sections.

Low crown
An inch or two above the nape of the neck.

Nape
The area where your hairline meets your neck.

Pancake
This is the act of pulling and stretching out the strands of a braid so as to create additional volume.

Round-brushing
Round brushes are good for creating curls. They also add grip while blow-drying so you are able to give the hair a sleeker finish.

Teasing
See back-combing.

Towel-drying
A method of drying the hair with a towel. When towel-drying, the hair should be squeezed through the towel, rather than rubbed, to avoid causing split ends.

Side fishtail bun, pages 36-37

CONTRIBUTOR CREDITS

Author's writing assistant
Cheyenne Folkert

All photography
Sara Bishop

Getty Images
(pages 121, 125)

Author's assistant
Emily Armijo

Models

Shelby Barnes
(pages 10–11, 38–39, 54–55, 70–71, 102–103)

Brianna Byars
(pages 88–89, 114–115)

Shireen Dooling
(pages 12–13, 72–73, 76–77, 86–87)

Cheyenne Folkert
(pages 16–17, 20–21, 36–37, 62–63, 108–109, 123)

Angela Gutierrez
(pages 6, 22–23, 40–41, 50–51, 64–65, 116–117)

Jasmine Jacobson
(pages 26–27, 60–61, 74–75, 104–105)

Mallory Jarvis
(pages 42–43, 52–53, 94–95)

Bryce May
(pages 28–29, 68–69, 90–91, 106–107)

Dominique Muscianese
(pages 14–15, 30–31, 48–49, 112–113)

Ashley Petty
(pages 80–81, 96–97, 110–111)

Alexia Poisot
(pages 18–19, 46–47, 82–83)

Jacque Stuard
(pages 24–25, 34–35, 44–45, 66–67)

Lacy Urban
(pages 58–59, 78–79, 92–93, 98–99)

WEBSITES

Jenny Strebe
theconfessionsofahairstylist.com

Other blogs
abeautifulmess.com

curlynikki.com

freckled-fox.com

hairandmakeupbysteph.com

hairromance.com

maneaddicts.com

missysue.com

thesmallthingsblog.comtwistmepretty.com

Training
Aveda Institutes
aveda.edu

Toni and Guy
Hairdressing Academytoniguy.edu

Vidal Sassoon Academy
sassoon-academy.com

Paul Mitchell
paulmitchell.edu

Regency Beauty Institute
regency.edu

Sharon Blain
sharonblain.com

Simple three-strand braid

INDEX

ACKNOWLEDGMENTS

This book has been an absolute dream to work on, thanks to my incredible support team, who have so kindly donated their talents and time to making it all happen.

The first of many thanks has to go to my supportive husband, Casey, whose constant love, patience, and encouragement has given me the strength to pursue my passion. You are my rock.

To my kids—your unconditional love means everything to me and helps me face the many challenges along the way. Thanks for always being my number-one fans.

A massive thank you to my photographer, Sara Bishop. You are an absolute star and super-talented woman. I was so grateful to have you in my corner, as always.

To my awesome rockstar editor, Angela Koo, who was an absolute joy to work with, and whose patience was outstanding. We couldn't have kept to the deadlines without you!

And lastly, a huge thank you to my writing assistant, Cheyenne Folkert, because without her patience during all of our photoshoots, and her putting my technical steps into beautiful words, this book just wouldn't be the same.